EMPOWERED JOURNEY THROUGH CANCER

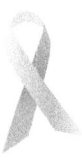

LEARN THE NITTY GRITTY TO PREPARE AND EXECUTE YOUR COMBAT PLAN

STEPHANIE CARROTHERS RPh

ISBN: 1492966282
ISBN 13: 9781492966289
Library of Congress Control Number: 2013920895
CreateSpace Independent Publishing Platform
North Charleston, South Carolina

Author's note

This book provides information to aid patients and caregivers when cancer is the diagnosis. Always follow the medical advice of your health-care professionals.

DEDICATIONS

To my husband, Michael: without your cancer diagnosis, this book would have never been written.

Dammit to hell.

To all those who have been diagnosed with cancer and the people that love them. If Michael and I could reach through this page and give you a great big hug, we would.

Contents

ACKNOWLEDGMENTS IX

FOREWORD XI

CHAPTER 1: THE DIAGNOSIS 1

CHAPTER 2: CHOOSING YOUR PLACE OF TREATMENT 13

CHAPTER 3: ASSEMBLE YOUR PROFESSIONAL TEAM 17

CHAPTER 4: THE FIRST ONCOLOGIST VISIT 31

CHAPTER 5: PORT AND PICC PLACEMENT 37

CHAPTER 6: PHYSICAL EFFECTS OF CANCER, CHEMOTHERAPY, AND TREATMENT 47

CHAPTER 7: MALNUTRITION KILLS 64

CHAPTER 8: EMOTIONAL EFFECTS 70

CHAPTER 9: CANCER PATIENT CAREGIVER 75

CHAPTER 10: OUTCOMES 80

CHAPTER 11: RIDING INTO THE SUNSET 84

SUPPLEMENTAL INFORMATION 87

REFERENCES 89

NOTES 91

ABOUT THE AUTHOR 93

ACKNOWLEDGMENTS

There are many people to thank for their help along the way. At the top of the list would be Michael's oncologist, Dr. Zyad Kafri. Because of your genuine caring nature and patience, we couldn't have been in better hands. Also, many thanks for your contribution to this book.

To Michael's boss, Tom Howley, for his compassion and understanding during Michael's chemotherapy treatment. Without your help, we would be in a totally different financial situation. There are not enough words of gratitude to express our thanks.

Additionally, I want to thank all the wonderful professionals who added valuable information to this book regarding their expertise. Thanks to:

Andrea Briefs-Ferris, RN, MHSA, CBPN-IC

Debra Averill, CPC

Suzanne Jermstad, MSN, FNP-BC, AOCNP, ACHPN, Oncology Nurse Practitioner

Lisa Currado, RN, OCN

And thanks to the fantastic nursing staff in the Van Elslander Cancer Center for your care; you made our many chemotherapy visits the best they could be.

A special thanks to Chris, RN, the midnight nurse at St. John Hospital; your extraordinary care will never be forgotten. Thanks for going to bat for us when we needed it.

FOREWORD

Confirming the news to Michael that the lump on his body was in fact cancer was life changing. Yet even though I was telling him that this was life threatening, I could see the strength of his spirit in his eyes. At that moment, I realized that Michael was no ordinary patient; he was a fighter. The battle facing him was cancer, specifically, large B-cell Non-Hodgkin's Lymphoma. In order to be well armed for this combat, he needed to be focused, determined, and emotionally stable. Fortunately, with the love of his supportive wife, Stephanie, Michael was able to adapt a strong-minded outlook and rise above the challenge. He was presented to St. John's lymphoma clinic, where he completed staging studies and had a bone marrow biopsy. He was enrolled in one of the St. John Providence Health System clinical trials for lymphoma. He successfully completed six cycles of standard chemotherapy, with complete remission of his disease. Afterward, he completed the experimental additional radio-immune therapy well, and he reacted positively to his experimental drug.

In order to successfully overcome cancer, one must be committed and consistent. Michael was exactly that. He attended every appointment, worked well with his treatment team, followed my instructions carefully, and did so while keeping a pleasant demeanor. His optimistic character coupled with his empowered attitude allowed him to win this battle. His story shines a realistic light on the different elements of cancer and helps anyone trotting down a similar path. Cancer presents emotional, physical, and mental setbacks, and this book serves as a comprehensive guide to push forward and persevere through it.

Zyad Kafri, MD
Hematologist/Oncologist
St. John Hematology-Oncology
St. John Providence Health System

"A journey of a thousand miles begins with a single step."
Lao-tzu

CHAPTER 1

THE DIAGNOSIS

We were lying in bed on a Sunday morning in late May when Michael said to me, "Hey, feel this lump that I have by my groin."

"What?" I asked.

He said, "Yeah, I've got this lump in the groin area."

"Well, how long have you had that?" I asked.

"I've had it for about a week," he said.

"What!?" I asked as I shot him a look.

"Yeah. Here, feel it. It's really hard."

I felt it and it felt like stone. It was very, very hard. I pushed on it and asked, "Does that hurt?"

"No."

So I pushed a little bit harder and asked, "Does that hurt?"

"No."

So, as I was feeling around, I noticed that it was probably about the size of a golf ball. I looked up at him with concern. "Oh, don't even go there," he said, "I don't even want to talk about that." With me working in oncology, he knew what was crossing my mind.

"All right," I said and felt around a little bit more. I kept pushing on the sides of it. "Does that hurt?"

"No."

"Well, you're going to have to go and get it checked out," I said.

"I don't think it's anything. I think it's just the hospital ID badge irritating it. I just moved the badge to the other side of my dress pants," he said.

"It's not from the badge irritating it," I said as I looked at him again with concern.

Both of us were thinking cancer, and I started getting sick to my stomach. I was thinking, "Oh my God, he's got some type of cancer." But I tried to keep calm, and thought, "Okay…it could be something else." I looked at him and said, "This is serious. You're going to have to get it checked out."

"I don't think so. I'll just wait to see if it goes away."

"No," I said. "You could have a hernia. And if it is a hernia, then you need to get it taken care of. It could get strangled, and that could lead to necrosis."

"What's necrosis?" Michael asked. "Talk in human people language here."

I explained, "Well, it's when the intestines that are sticking through the abdominal wall actually get strangled and die. When they die off, that is necrosis. If the intestines die off, then you'll need to have a poop bag, and I ain't changing no poop bag." We both laughed. "So you better go get it looked at."

"All right, I'll go in."

So he went into the doctor's office. I wasn't able to go with him because I had to work. The doctor scheduled him for an ultrasound, and a couple days later the ultrasound came back. It was not a hernia.

"Okay," I said. "If it's not a hernia, what does that doctor think it is?"

"He thinks it might be an infection."

"An infection?! If it was an infection, it would be swollen, yes, but it would also be tender, like when your lymph nodes in your neck are tender when you have an infection. That thing you have is as hard as a rock, and you said it doesn't hurt."

He said, "Well, he gave me this antibiotic to take. So I am going to take it and see how I do."

I was upset. I said, "You need to have that thing biopsied if it's not a hernia."

He said, "The doctor just said to take the antibiotic for ten days and to go and enjoy our trip to Florida. He will see me when I get back."

We were supposed to go to Florida a few days later. However, I threw my back out and was unable to even really walk. So we canceled the trip.

About five days into the antibiotic treatment, the lump was not getting any better; the swelling had not gone down one bit. I started getting extremely anxious. I told Michael, "We have to have this thing biopsied. We have to see what this thing is. We can't just let this go on indefinitely."

Michael said, "We could just wait and see."

"I am not the 'wait-and-see' kind of girl," I said. "We need to go in." So I made him make another appointment to see the doctor. In a few days, we went in and I expressed my concerns about the lump not getting any better. If this was an infection, the antibiotic was not helping at all. I told the doctor that we needed to do something. I believed Michael needed to have a biopsy to make sure it wasn't anything serious.

The doctor said that it was probably just an infection. Then he told us a story about how when he was in college he had had a swollen gland in his neck that was biopsied. It turned out to be nothing.

I was so angry. Here he was talking about himself. I could care less about what his history was! We weren't here to discuss him. We were here for Michael.

Looking back, I am sure that he was trying to assure me that he believed it was probably just an infection. But at the time, all I could think about was the possibility of Michael having cancer and that we were doing nothing about it.

Because I was upset that we weren't doing a biopsy and that my fiancé might have cancer, I pulled out the oncology pharmacist card. "Did you know that I work in oncology?" I asked.

He looked up from his note-taking.

"I am a pharmacist at one of the hospitals in the area. I make up all the IV chemotherapy for the patients." I waited out the long pause. "I think we should do a biopsy." The eyebrows of the resident in the room rose.

At that point, he said to keep taking the antibiotic but, if something else was to come up, to come in right away.

I was so angry and upset leaving the doctor's office. As we were walking to the car, Michael said to me, "You're upset; you're angry."

"You're damn right I'm angry," I said. "Antibiotics, come on! This is ridiculous. I'm so angry right now I could spit nails." I said many other things, which have since then been censored out of this account. We got in the car, and I said to him, "You need to switch doctors."

"Are you calling my doctor a quack?"

"I'm not calling him a quack. I'm just saying that he is not listening."

We left there with Michael still being on antibiotics and still not having the biopsy. It was now the middle of June.

When I went back to work the next day, I told the nurse manager of the cancer center about our doctor visit. She tried to comfort me by saying that we always think the worst because we work in oncology. "Most of the time it is not cancer," she said. "Statistically speaking, it probably is not cancer." Then I thought that maybe I was too hard on the doctor. Maybe I should relax. I told her that I heard what she was saying, but I still had a sinking feeling that it was cancer.

About a week after we went to see the doctor, Michael got another lump on the same side about two inches below the first lump. He showed it to me on the Sunday of the following weekend. I told Michael that he had to go in on Monday and demand to have a biopsy. By this time, it was the end of June. Now he had two lumps, although the second lump was obviously not as big as the first one.

So Michael went in and finally got a surgical referral for a biopsy. When he met with the surgeon, the surgeon told Michael that he had three choices. He could do nothing, but Michael quickly interjected, "Stephanie would never go for that." Then the surgeon said that they could biopsy it. The third option was to take it out. Michael said there was no way he was going to have it removed. So we would have to compromise and do a biopsy.

The biopsy was done the last week of June. We were told to expect the results in about a week to ten days. The surgeon told Michael that the results might be delayed because of the holiday. On the fifth of July, Michael called to say that he wanted to meet me after work. I wasn't even thinking that the results were in. We met at my house in Royal Oak and sat down on the sofa. "I didn't really want to tell you what I wanted to talk to you about until I saw you," he said. He looked at me, and I gripped his hand a bit harder. "The biopsy came back, and it is cancer. It's a lymphoma."

As I sat there, a bit numb and upset from the news, he said, "Don't cry, don't cry." I knew that if I cried he probably would too. I tried to be strong and switch gears to my professional role.

Michael pulled a piece of paper from his pocket and read, "He says it is a DLBC lymphoma. What can you tell me about this? What are my chances of beating this?"

We talked for a while about what lymphoma is and the course of chemo treatment that is usually recommended to fight it. I told him that when I went to work the next day, I would find out all the information I possibly could. Also, since Michael works for St. John, I told him that I would find out who was the best oncologist in the St. John Health System for him to see. Where I work, at St. Joseph Mercy Oakland (SJMO), we have a group of physicians that works for both SJMO and St. John.

GET YOUR DOCTOR TO LISTEN

The one message to take away from this is that you know your body. You have to trust your gut and get your doctor to listen. If your doctor is not listening to you, you have the right to fire your doctor. There have been many cases where people have gone in and had lumps, only to have the doctor say, "It's just a cyst. We don't need a biopsy on that." There have also been cases where the doctor says that it's a cyst, only for it to be biopsied and turn out to be cancer.

So if you're not getting the answers that you want, seek another opinion. If that person doesn't give you the answer you want, seek another opinion. Get someone who is going to listen to you and who's going to be on your side.

You have to be your own advocate. In order to be your own advocate, you have to have some knowledge to be successful. Having worked as a pharmacist in a hospital health-care system since the mid-1990s, I knew many of the answers to the questions that most people would have. However, if I didn't know the answer to a question, I knew which health-care professional could give it to me. If you have never worked in health care, you most likely don't even know where to begin, let alone the questions to ask. Because this diagnosis requires a steep learning curve, I will cover what you will most likely encounter along with the "answers" you will be looking for and/or the professional to ask. Additionally, the experiences Michael and I encountered while navigating our own journey are layered within. Let us begin.

ASSEMBLE YOUR PERSONAL TEAM

The first step in becoming your own advocate is to start assembling your personal team. This begins with your inner circle of family, friends, and neighbors. These are the people that you're going to have to count on to help you through this whole process. So what Michael and I decided to do was to have a family meeting. We made dinner for everyone. Then, after we were done eating, we broke the news to the entire family. As I was explaining the events that led up to Michael's diagnosis, his sister, Cheri, was starting to cry. All the emotions were welling up inside of me as I saw how hard it was on her. I knew it would be hard on everyone, so I tried to stay focused on the factual information while telling them the news.

We decided to tell everyone this way so there would be no misinformation given second- and third-hand. Everybody would be on the same page. Also, at that moment, we could enlist the help of our family.

Your family and friends will most likely feel overwhelmed, but they are also going to want to help in any way they can. Giving them tasks allows them to be part of the process of "doing something" for you. It makes them feel useful, and it gets the things done that you're unable to do during this time.

Before going into this meeting, you need to assess your whole situation. This way you can more thoroughly plan your strategy. In our case, Michael and I were engaged, but we were living in separate houses. So we had two houses to maintain, and I wasn't going to be able to be at his house all the time. He needed people to come and check in on him when I wasn't there, especially when I was working, and at this time, I was working full time. That was our situation. We were going to need a lot of support from his family. During the meeting we covered the following topics:

- Taking Michael to appointments, if I could not get time off from work
- The possibility of surgery
- Assistance if Michael got sick (as well as the issue of family members not visiting if they were sick)
- The possibility of hospitalization
- Education of the family on lymphoma

After a cancer diagnosis, life will continue on around you. You will have to formulate a game plan in order to clarify what you need to accomplish in all areas of your life. This is going to be a marathon and not a sprint. You need to enlist the help of others.

STRATEGIC AREAS

Finances

You need to figure out the bills. If the person who is diagnosed is the one who does the finances, the other person is going to need to take over that responsibility.

Food

Consider having your family and friends cook for you. A really good way to do this is to provide options for them. Don't just ask them to bring "something" over. Rather, ask them to bring you chicken soup or chicken casserole or some other specific dishes. Give them options for the kinds of meals they can cook that you would eat.

Children

You also have to think about care for your children, as well as how they will be affected by the diagnosis. Following is a list of categories pertaining to child care:
- School: including transportation, homework, and events related to school
- Activities
- Telling your children the diagnosis

Emotional Support

You may want to enlist the help of a psychologist, psychiatrist, or your clergy. The diagnosis will affect everyone; however, you may want to especially consider how it will affect your children. Children react in different ways to troubling news, and it is possible that you might witness your child acting out, behaving very clingy, or becoming depressed and reclusive. So you may want to think about setting up sessions for them early on.

Household Chores

Household chores, both inside and outside the house, will still need to be done. When figuring out what needs to be done, it makes sense to be as thorough as possible. Does your grass need to be cut? Does your snow need to be plowed? Can someone else come and clean? Are there any small repairs that need to be done? Can someone coordinate all the tasks that need to be done?

This is one area that I strongly urge you to get help with. You are going to be exhausted throughout this process. Not only does chemotherapy make a person tired, but the emotional drain of the diagnosis also will exhaust everyone involved.

The Job

These questions will help you determine how to adjust your financial situation to these new circumstances.

- Who provides the main source of financial support for your family?
- What type of boss do you have, someone strict or easygoing?
- Will your boss allow you to take time off from work?
- Is your boss flexible?
- Would you be able to work from home?

In Michael's case, his boss was extremely understanding and flexible. He always allowed Michael to take the day off of work if necessary, and he also let Michael work from home after chemo treatments.

However, my boss was not as flexible. When I tried to get time off for Michael's first appointment, there was simply no one available to take over my responsibilities. Out of the three people who usually covered for my position, one was on vacation, another was having a party for her niece, and the third had not covered the position in over a year, so the manager would not allow it. I was extremely upset. I told Michael that I wanted to go to his first oncology visit, but Michael understood that there was no one to cover for me. I wanted to call in sick, but Michael dissuaded me from doing this because he knew that in the end it would be my patients who would suffer. Then he made me laugh by quoting *Star Trek*'s Mr. Spock: "The needs of the many outweigh the needs of the one." I was still upset, but nevertheless, I went into work, and he went alone.

All I could think about that day was that I wasn't there for him and that I had no idea what was being discussed. To this day, I still regret not having gone to the first appointment. The first appointment is when the diagnosis is confirmed, additional testing is discussed, and the game plan is laid out. It is crucial to go to the first appointment.

Michael's oncologist, Dr. Kafri, was extremely understanding. He set up an extra doctor's appointment. This way, he could go over all the information with me that he had already discussed with Michael.

Your marital status with your partner can have a significant impact on how easily you can make the practical arrangements for treatment.

- Are you and your partner married?
- Can you apply for Family Medical Leave Act (FMLA)?

When I approached my boss later on, I told him that in the future, I was going to want to take some time off for Michael's chemotherapy appointments. I got a lot of resistance from management about this, and they refused to guarantee me time off for Michael's treatment. At the time we were engaged and not yet married, so we decided to push the wedding forward and do it immediately. This way, we would qualify for family medical leave, and I could be there for him. Dr. Kafri filled out the necessary medical paperwork, specifying that I should be granted time off for any reason relating to Michael's diagnosis, foreseen or unforeseen.

Diagnosis-Related Appointments

The person with the diagnosis may require help getting to appointments. There can be a battery of tests and other checkups such as:

- Physician appointments
- Lab draws
- Chemotherapy appointments
- Medical personnel–administered shots
- Radiation appointments
- Follow-up testing, including PET, CT, and MUGA scans

Enlist the help of your family, friends, and neighbors to get you through this time. Everyone in the core unit of the family is going to want to pitch in. People love to help; it makes them feel useful and allows them to feel like they are doing something important. Help them help you, any way they can.

If your family and friends are not in your area, you can still build a team. Start by looking for community resources. Right off the bat, a good one to sign up for is Meals on Wheels; this way, food can be provided. Also, check in with the cancer resource center at your place of treatment to see what services it has to offer. Many churches also have outreach programs.

"A good decision is based on knowledge and not on numbers."
Plato

CHAPTER 2

CHOOSING YOUR PLACE OF TREATMENT

Choosing a place for Michael to receive his treatment was straightforward because he works for, and has insurance through, the St. John Health Care System. So in order to stay "in network" where his medical bills would be covered at the highest percentage rate, he decided to go there for treatment. If he were to have chosen another hospital system, he would have had to pay the "out of network" costs. So we decided that it would be best for us to stay within the St. John system. However, if he had *needed* to go out of network, we would have, but fortunately there wasn't any reason to change his place of treatment.

If you have no insurance restrictions and you can choose where you want to go, what are the criteria you should use? Understand that the size of the treatment place can dictate its strengths and limitations. With this in mind, you can determine the best fit.

Large institutions have more resources and a greater number of clinical trials available. Because of this, they are usually on the cutting edge of new treatments. Additionally, they do bone marrow transplants (BMTs) procedures and post care. Because they are large, they treat a greater number of patients. Therefore, one of the biggest limitations you may find is the wait time you could encounter. Also, people who prefer a lot of one-on-one time may feel their need of personalized care is not being met.

On the opposite end of the spectrum is a very small hospital or doctor's office. The major benefit that a smaller size facility or practitioner can provide is individual one-on-one time. Because cancer is a very stressful diagnosis, this can be a great comfort. The major drawbacks are there may not be trials available that you would qualify for, or they might not offer the ancillary staff that you might need. The ancillary support staff is detailed in chapter three.

A medium size institution has fewer numbers of patients than a larger institution, which may translate into less wait time and possibly more one-on-one time. Also, they have trials available and ancillary staff to assist you. I would categorize the place where Michael received his treatment as a medium size institution. Michael qualified for a trial to receive Zevalin®, which is a radioactive isotope given in combination with another medication. He received this after the traditional chemotherapy treatment for lymphoma was completed.

When examining different health-care systems, ask about the additional services they have available. These services should include:

1. Financial services: See if the institution has a financial navigator on staff. This person can help with the high costs of treatment.
2. Physical services: Some places have extra services available for physical care. These may include massage-therapy, the Look Good Feel Better program, and wig or prostheses information.
3. Emotional support groups
4. A library or resource center: The on-site library or resource center is a great place you can go to find information, support materials, and personalized help. When you have access to the resources, you will see that there are national and local support systems in place for patients. For example, in our area, there is a house-cleaning service available for free for patients receiving chemotherapy.

5. On-site pharmacist-staffed pharmacy: If the facility is medium-sized or larger, it will usually have its own pharmacy dedicated solely to the compounding of chemotherapy and staffed by at least one pharmacist. Because the pharmacy compounds the medication specifically to your dose according to the orders your physician writes, having an on-site pharmacy is going to significantly reduce your wait time. The pharmacist's job is to review orders, compound or oversee trained technicians in the compounding of medications, and dispense them to the nursing staff. This close contact between staff members also provides additional security and safety. The pharmacist is also available as a resource for questions that you may have about chemotherapy, its side effects, and your support medications. Note: Be aware that doctor's offices that give chemotherapy are not required by law to staff a pharmacist for the review of orders or the overseeing of a technician for the compounding of medication. Additionally, they do not have to adhere to the strict "aseptic" guidelines that hospital systems do.

"Individual commitment to a group effort—that's what makes a team work, a company work, a society work, a civilization work."
Vince Lombardi

CHAPTER 3

ASSEMBLE YOUR PROFESSIONAL TEAM

Once you've decided where you want to be treated, begin assembling your professional team. These professionals are there to help you throughout your medical journey. Ask for the help you need.

THE ONCOLOGIST

The first person you should hire for your professional team is an oncologist. Search for someone who specializes in your type of cancer. Not every cancer type has its own specialized field; however, if your type of cancer has a specialist, I would highly recommend that you go to see that physician.

When Michael was diagnosed with lymphoma, I knew that there were oncologists who specialized in lymphoma (hematology oncology). So when I went into work the next day, I asked Dr. Goodman whom Michael should see in the St. John system. Dr. Goodman is an oncologist who works for both the St. Joseph Mercy Oakland (SJMO) system (where I work) and the St. John system (where Michael works). So I knew she would know whom he should go to see in the St. John system. She recommended that we see Dr. Al-Katib.

I called Michael and told him he should call this doctor's office and get an appointment set up right away. When Michael called the office, Dr. Al-Katib was not taking new patients. However, his partner, Dr. Kafri, was. Michael called on a Friday, and the office was able to squeeze him in on the next Monday. Knowing he had a positive biopsy for diffuse large B-cell lymphoma, (DLBC Lymphoma), I was relieved that he was going to be seen quickly.

I will say this again: if you have the opportunity to see a specialist in the type of cancer you have been diagnosed with, I would highly recommend that you do this.

For further clarification and understanding of the oncologist's role on your team, I posed the following questions to Dr. Zyad Kafri.

What area of oncology do you specialize in?

All types of lymphoma in addition to lung and colorectal cancer.

What makes that specialty unique?
- The disease (cancer) is life threatening.
- Treatment usually requires ongoing chemotherapy.
- There are short-term and long-term treatment complications related to chemotherapy toxicity.
- The journey through treatment is a life- changing experience for most patients.
- It has social impacts; both work and family life are affected.
- I build a long-lasting relationship with the patient.

What are the most common side effects of chemotherapy you see? How are they managed?
1. Nausea and vomiting: can be prevented by giving medications to prepare patients before and after chemotherapy
2. Fatigue: management is usually supportive
3. Hair loss: does not happen with every regimen. Hair will grow back after stopping chemotherapy. Some (female) patients may choose to use the "ice hat." It can

help, but does not necessarily work for everyone. They are also pricey and labor intensive.

4. Neuropathy (numbness, tingling, and/or pain in the extremities): results from some chemotherapeutic agents. Reducing chemotherapy doses or using medications, such as Gabapentin, to reduce the sensation may help with this.

How can the patient and/or caregiver take an active role in the patient's care plan?

- Through better understanding of treatment plan requirements
- By taking notes during clinic visits when the treating team is giving instructions
- By doing their own personal research and reading that will help them understand why they are taking chemotherapy and what to expect from the therapy
- Caregivers can help patients keep their appointments and help them at home with their daily needs

What instructions do you give to patients that you would like to stress as VERY IMPORTANT?

- If you trust your treating doctor, you need to follow all of his or her treatment recommendations.
- Never hesitate to question your treating team about the rationale behind doing things that you don't understand.
- Communication and compliance are the keys to treatment success and patient satisfaction.

When should patients consider getting a second opinion?

1. If they have rare disease
2. If they want validation of the proposed treatment plan
3. If they have difficulty understanding their disease or prognosis
4. If they want to explore other treatment options
5. If they did not connect well with their oncologists
6. If they are seeking clinical trials

Nurse Practitioner or Physician Assistant

Another person that you may see while you're in the oncologist's office is a nurse practitioner (NP) or physician assistant (PA). The nurse practitioner and physician assistant work with the oncologist. They generally will see patients for routine visits and follow-ups. Many offices have them.

NURSE NAVIGATOR

These professionals can be very helpful if they are available. They help patients "navigate" through the system. Often, "nurse navigators" help patients with a specific cancer type. For example, at SJMO we have a nurse navigator for breast cancer, Andrea Briefs-Ferris, RN, MHSA, CBPN-IC.

I asked Andrea if she could share some of her expertise with me through a series of questions.

1. What is a nurse navigator?

The role of "patient navigator" was conceived by Dr. Harold Freeman in 1990. He is an oncologic surgeon who, while working at Harlem City Hospital, noticed the disparity in treatment for minority groups with breast cancer and developed the concept of the navigation role to help bridge the gap in care.

At St. Joseph Mercy Oakland, the breast cancer nurse navigator provides newly diagnosed patients with guidance and support throughout their treatment and into survivorship or end-of-life, as the case may be. The nurse navigator assesses each case for any barriers hindering the completion of the treatment plan and attempts to make the treatment experience as smooth as possible for patients.

Treatment barriers may occur in the realms of:

- Finances: especially for the underinsured or the uninsured
- Communication: difficulty understanding language differences (including jargon)
- Health systems: navigating the health system, including understanding appointment systems and managing multiple doctors' appointments
- Patient psychology: fear and distrust of the medical system or of the diagnosis
- Transportation

Navigators assist patients with everything from the emotional to the logistical so that patients understand medical information and their treatment options.

2. How is it that you help patients?

Based on the barriers assessment and the patient's needs and wishes, "action steps" will be determined. They can include:

- Referring the patient to the oncology financial navigator (who also provides info about food banks, utilities, other help, etc.)
- Determining if community resources can satisfy any of the patient's needs—most often, to provide wigs and prostheses
- Finding support for the patient either by individual consultation or via the monthly support group
- Recommending Look Good Feel Better education for skin, scalp, and nail care during treatment
- Attending physician appointments to take notes or to be a "second set of ears"
- Educating patients regarding their illness and treatment options

3. What additional services are provided to aid breast cancer patients?

Other services include psych support, nutritional education, and genetics counseling. We assist patients by getting financial grants from grassroots organizations to help pay for their living expenses.

GENETIC COUNSELOR

Depending on your type of cancer, you may benefit from genetics counseling. At SJMO, one of our genetics counselors is Suzanne Jermstad, MSN, FNP-BC, AOCNP, ACHPN, and an oncology nurse practitioner.

I asked Suzanne to share information about genetic counseling.

1. Why should one do genetic screening?

Genetic information helps to determine which individuals are at a higher risk for developing cancer. This is a powerful tool in terms of early detection. Individuals with identified genetic mutations have the power to change their future by following the recommended guidelines to reduce overall cancer risk.

2. What is the role of a genetic counselor?

The role of the genetic counselor is to gather information about the patient based on personal and family history. The counselor helps determine which patients and family members are at a higher risk for certain genetic mutations. In addition, the genetic counselor generally participates in discussions about the benefits and limitations of genetic testing, as well as about recommendations for going forward based on the test results. Typically, genetic counselors work on a team with a physician or NP who can provide clinical expertise.

3. Which cancers have a genetic link?

The most common cancers that have a genetic link are breast, ovarian, endometrial, and colon cancer. The genes identified are BRCA1 and BRCA2. Mutations in either of these genes increase an individual's risk of developing breast and ovarian cancer. In addition, there are other genes that are typically studied in families with a history of colon cancer.

These genetic tests help to identify families with Lynch syndrome or HNPCC. Lynch syndrome families have an increased risk of colon, endometrial, and ovarian cancer.

4. Who should be tested?

Those who should be tested include:
- anyone under the age of fifty with breast, ovarian, colon, or endometrial cancer
- anyone with a personal history of breast cancer at any age with two first-degree relatives under fifty who have been diagnosed with breast or ovarian cancer
- anyone with colon cancer under fifty or with two first-degree relatives under fifty
- anyone with breast cancer and Ashkenazi Jewish ancestry

5. What is involved in the testing?

Testing usually involves meeting with a genetic counselor for discussion and determination of criteria for testing. Most insurance companies require pre-testing counseling with a certified genetic expert. The tests are routine blood draws.

6. Does insurance cover it?

Most insurance companies cover testing for those who meet established criteria. These criteria can be located on the NCCN (National Comprehensive Cancer Network) website. The tests themselves are currently quite expensive, so it is important for patients to call their insurance carrier to make sure that genetics counseling and testing is a covered benefit.

FINANCIAL NAVIGATOR

At SJMO, our financial navigator is Debra Averill, CPC. Here she offers some helpful information on the role of financial navigators and the services they provide.

1. What is a financial navigator?

A financial navigator assists patients who are uninsured or underinsured with obtaining additional coverage when needed for a better patient outcome.

If a patient is enrolled in Medicare A and B only and receives chemotherapy and/or radiation, the patient will be responsible for a 20 percent co-pay fee. To help cover the costs, we would look at enrolling this patient in a Medigap secondary plan.

For patients with private insurance and a large deductible or co-pay for medication, we would review the option of a possible secondary (Medicaid) and/or a pharmaceutical co-pay assistance program.

For those uninsured, we screen all patients for available coverage programs. We also would check for possible Social Security Disability enrollment.

2. How do you help patients find coverage for their medications?

I use www.needymeds.com. You can search by brand or generic name. If I cannot find a program for the medication, I will go to the pharmaceutical website to see if they have any programs available for the patient that were not listed.

3. What is the first thing you look at?

The first thing I review is the patient's coverage and the course of treatment. I contact the insurance company for co-payment and deductible information. This will define the patient's needs.

4. What information does the patient need to bring for his or her appointment?

If insured, I will need a copy of their insurance card, driver's license, a current bank statement, and proof of all household income. If uninsured, I will require the same documents with the exception of insurance card.

5. If a patient has insurance, can he or she still be helped by a financial navigator?

Absolutely. We can look for specific grants available for their co-pays and deductibles. The patient may also be eligible for Medicaid secondary to assist with the co-pays and deductibles. The patient could also be eligible for Social Security Disability.

6. With the Affordable Care Act (often referred to as Obamacare), will patients receive better coverage, less coverage, or about the same amount?

The Affordable Care Act will allow patients with preexisting conditions to qualify for insurance without penalty or time delay. Currently under Medicaid restrictions, patients who have a savings of over $2,000 per single person, or $3,000 per married couple, cannot apply for coverage. With the Affordable Care Act, these restrictions do not apply.

7. How can pharmaceutical companies help cover costs?

Pharmaceutical companies can supply the medication for free or assist with a co-pay program specific to the medication. Additionally, some tests can be covered, including genetic testing like Oncotype DX testing for breast, prostate, and colon cancer.[1]

EMPLOYER OFFERED HEALTHCARE SAVINGS OR REIMBURSEMENT ACCOUNTS

Michael had good insurance through his job working for a health-care system. However, even with good insurance, he encountered additional expenses. Fortunately, he had enrolled in the health-care savings account through work, which he was able to use for these expenses. Health-care savings accounts or health-care reimbursement accounts can cover out-of-pocket costs, such as physician visit co-pays, medication co-pays, testing, laboratory tests, biopsies, surgeries, and more. Check to see if your employer offers one of these programs.

ONCOLOGY NURSE

At SJMO, one of our oncology nurses is Lisa Currado, RN, OCN. I asked Lisa to share some of her expertise with us about her frontline experience.

---

[1]   See http://www.breastcancer.org/symptoms/testing/types/oncotype_dx.

1. What is the role of the oncology nurse?

The oncology nurse's role has many facets: patient assessment, patient education, coordination of care with other members of the health-care team, direct patient care, symptom management, and supportive care.

Assessment means physically assessing the patient before, during, and after treatments. Assessment also includes evaluating the patient's emotional status and past medical history, as well as his or her understanding of the disease process and the proposed treatment.

2. Do you have any extra training or credentialing?

There is no mandatory national credentialing for oncology nursing or chemotherapy in particular. Each institution should have its own written policies for chemotherapy certification and the administration of chemotherapy (for all routes of administration).

Although certification as an oncology nurse (OCN) is voluntary, institutions prefer RNs to have it. Recertification is required every four years to maintain the credential, which is currently done either by retesting or presenting one hundred CEUs (continuing education credits). A nurse should have worked the equivalent of two and half years in oncology before applying for certification.

At SJMO, RNs are required to attend a chemotherapy class, followed by check-off by an experienced RN, before administering chemotherapy.

3. What are some of the instructions you give to all patients regardless of their primary cancer diagnosis?

I explain the side effects of chemotherapy, both specifically and generally, and the "self-care" activities one can use to reduce their severity. I also show them how to look for signs and symptoms of infection, and I tell them who and when to call with problems and/or questions. I also review their expected treatment outcomes with them. Overall, I emphasize the general importance of communication with all members of the health-care team, including MDs, NPs and RNs.

4. What is the biggest pitfall that patients encounter during treatment?

The biggest pitfall is miscommunication or lack of communication. This can be a result of the health-care team not providing enough information or presenting information at the inappropriate level for the patient to understand it. This can also be a result of patients not informing the nurses or physicians of problems or concerns they may be experiencing. I believe every person needs to understand that there are no "dumb questions."

ONCOLOGY PHARMACIST

This is the service that I provide at SJMO. An oncology pharmacist reviews the physician orders. Pharmacists make, or supervise trained technicians that make, your chemotherapy. They are available to answer questions about chemotherapy and other support medications. One of the recommendations that I always give to patients is that they should not to take any herbal supplements or over-the-counter medications without talking to their oncologist first. Some of these can have adverse interactions with the chemotherapy.

NUTRITIONIST

Most hospitals have nutritionists on staff, and you can request to speak to one, if you so choose. During Michael's first chemotherapy infusion, when we were in the St. John chemo-infusion room, the nutritionist came in and asked if we had any questions for him. Nutritionists have a lot of resources available for you if you want them.

PSYCHOLOGIST/PSYCHIATRIST

Psychologists and psychiatrists are available for outpatient support in many health-care systems. If you would like to take advantage of their services, you can be referred to one of them to help you cope with the diagnosis, as well as with day-to-day life.

SUPPORT GROUPS

Most facilities also have support groups available. These groups will usually meet at the hospital or in the cancer resource center. There are groups for both patient support and caregiver support.

"We are not preparing for the world we live in—we are preparing for the world we find ourselves in."
Michael Mabee

CHAPTER 4

THE FIRST ONCOLOGIST VISIT

Missing Michael's first two oncology visits was something that I was extremely upset about. Luckily, Michael's oncologist, Dr. Kafri, was very accommodating by going over the information again in an additional physician appointment I could attend. At the appointment, Dr. Kafri explained the lymphoma type that Michael had, as well as the staging, the goals of treatment, the course of treatment, the percentages for remission, and other options, including the possibility for Michael to be in a trial.

THE FIRST VISIT

The first visit is usually to confirm the findings of the surgeon or primary care physician, as well as, setting up additional testing. Additional testing will help determine the extent to which the cancer has spread. The way that cancer spreads is classified in four stages.

Stage 0: The cancer is in the place of origin and has not spread to other tissues. The mass is removed by surgery if possible.

Stage I: The cancer has spread to nearby tissues but not the lymph nodes. This is often referred to as early diagnosis.

Stage II and III: The cancer has spread to nearby tissues and lymph nodes.

Stage IV: The cancer has spread to other organs or parts of the body. This is referred to as metastatic cancer.

The stage helps determine the course of treatment. Additional testing that Michael had after his first visit were CT scan, PET scan, MUGA scan, Bone Marrow Biopsy, and blood work.

During your first visit to the oncologist, you are going to have many emotions running through you. You might experience some or all of these:

- Nervousness
- Anxiety
- Confusion
- Anger
- Denial
- Feeling lost
- Shock
- Fatigue
- Uncertainty

Michael happened to be feeling extremely fatigued before he was diagnosed. However, you might have a completely different response and show up to your appointment with an "I'm-going-to-kick-cancer's-ass" attitude, turning on your "Rocky" persona against the disease.

Considering that you will be experiencing a variety of emotions and because this will all be uncharted territory, it is highly recommended that you *bring a voice recorder*. The doctor will not mind being recorded. In fact, he or she will probably encourage it. If the physician does mind, this should be a red flag for you. Perhaps it might serve you well to find another oncologist. The purpose of the voice recorder is to remember everything *for you* because you probably won't be able to. If you bring one, you will be able to go back and listen to the whole exchange and to go over things that maybe you thought you understood but didn't really, as well as get access to the things you couldn't remember. Whatever the case may be, the recorder will save the information for you.

You are also going to need to bring a **list of your current medications including over-the-counter medications, vitamin and herbal supplements**.

You will need to present your full medical history. Your history can affect the course of treatment and/or the medications prescribed.

THE FOLLOW-UP VISIT

After all the tests have been run and the results are in, you will have a follow-up visit to go over the results. The oncologist will have the staging, prognosis, and treatment plan for you. Remember to bring your voice recorder to this appointment. There is going to be a lot of information in this meeting. If there is terminology or medical jargon used that you don't understand, ask the oncologist to explain it further. We had told our family about Michael's diagnosis before the follow-up visit. Michael's mom went with him to this appointment, as I was still having difficulty getting time off work.

You will want to make sure these questions are covered in your follow-up appointment.

- What is my exact diagnosis? For example, Michael's diagnosis was diffuse large B-cell lymphoma (DLBC lymphoma).
- What stage am I? What does that mean? Michael was a stage III lymphoma. That meant it had spread to lymph nodes above and below the belly button. However, it was not in the bone marrow or other organs.
- What are my treatment options?

Many times treatment is straightforward. The cancer type, the staging, and the medical history of the cancer patient usually dictate the course of treatment. Make sure you know the answers to these questions:

- Do I need surgery?
- Am I going to receive chemotherapy?
- Am I going to receive radiation?
- Am I going to receive both chemo and radiation?
- Are there trials available that I qualify for?

Michael qualified for a trial. If you do sign up for a trial, just be aware that there will be more paperwork and more follow-ups. There are no costs for the patient to be enrolled in a trial, and sometimes you receive the drug(s) for free.

So if you do get chemotherapy, you're going to want to know what drugs you are going to be receiving, the frequency of your treatment, the length treatment (number of cycles), and the time it will take to infuse all the medications.

Michael had his chemotherapy regimen on one day every three weeks, and he was going to receive six cycles (six treatments), each of which lasted about six hours in the chemotherapy infusion center. There are multiple regimens that can be prescribe, it is determined on what type of cancer is being treated and at what stage it's in.

Ask about the side effects of chemotherapy and how to manage them. What medications are going to be prescribed for the side effects?

If you get the list of chemotherapy medications they are going to prescribe, there is a fantastic website you can use to get a ton of information. The website is www.chemocare.com. This website explains all the side effects of the specific drugs that you will be taking, and it also has some managing tips for each specific medication.

Because of the need for further testing, appointments, and possible surgery, the first chemotherapy usually begins about three to six weeks after the initial diagnosis. You may feel anxious about waiting this long before getting started. Typically, cancer patients feel like they need to start tomorrow. But realize you have a window of time to formulate a plan and get another opinion if necessary. After testing, appointments and port placement, Michael received his first chemotherapy four weeks after diagnosis.

Additional questions about treatment include:
- Who should I contact if I have a problem after hours?
- What are the specific conditions that require I go to the emergency room?
- When will we recheck the progress of the treatment to see if it's working?
- Should I get a port or PICC line placed? (There is more information on port and PICC line placements in chapter 5.)

Questions regarding sex and chemotherapy include:
- Should I abstain from sex when getting chemo?
- If so, for how long?
- Should I use a condom?

Usually we tell our patients to wait about seventy-two hours after treatment, but you should check with your oncologist. It just depends on what kind of therapy you're getting and what your doctor recommends.

Ask to visit the chemo-infusion room before you receive chemotherapy. This will give you an idea of how it is set up and what's available to you.
- Do they have wireless Internet?
- Do they have televisions?
- Do they have computers?
- Can you bring your electronic devices to pass the time?
- If your infusion will be long, do they have food available?
- Do they have a food service that comes in for you to purchase food?
- Do you need to bring something to eat?

Be sure to have some type of journal to document and organize everything in one place. Write down all the information you need for quick reference. Additionally, Chapter 4 is available as a free download at the website: http://www.stephaniecarrothers. com/.

"Take calculated risks. That is quite different from being rash."
George S. Patton

CHAPTER 5

Port and PICC Placement

PORT PLACEMENT

When Michael saw Dr. Kafri for his initial visit, he recommended that Michael get a port placed for his chemotherapy. A port for delivering chemotherapy is a small device that is inserted surgically underneath the skin. The port has a reservoir with a tube, often referred to as a catheter, attached to it. The catheter is threaded through a large vein near your collar bone so the tip of the catheter is just above the heart. Michael's port catheter was placed in his upper chest and threaded into his veins with the catheter tip ending near his heart. The chemotherapy and other medications are delivered from the IV line into the port reservoir, through the catheter, and into the bloodstream close to the heart. Since the port is under the skin, a needle like device is used to deliver fluids from the IV line to the port reservoir.

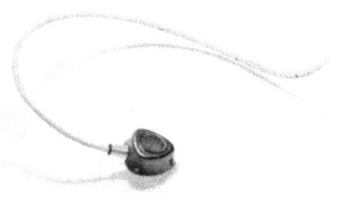

$$\text{PORT}^2$$

REASONS FOR PORT PLACEMENTS

Michael got a port because his chemotherapy could be very caustic and cause phlebitis. Phlebitis is inflammation of the veins. This is one reason why you might need to get a port. Another reason ports are used is because some chemotherapy can be given only through ports. In such cases, it cannot be given peripherally through an IV line in the arm.

Additionally, if you are going to have several chemotherapy cycles (at least four) over several months, the doctor may recommend getting a port. Some people have veins that are very difficult to access. Mine are small, difficult to access, and refuse to give blood most times. If I ever had to receive chemo, I would definitely need a port; it would be time-consuming to try to insert an IV line in me. Besides being difficult, if the nurse cannot get good IV access, it could delay therapy.

Getting a port placed is an outpatient surgical procedure. I was unable to take Michael to the port-placement procedure because of work, so his brother Bob took him that day. He went in, got it placed, and was home the same day. The surgery left about a two-inch scar on his upper chest.

If the patient is having another surgical procedure, such as a mastectomy for breast cancer, the surgeon may place the port at the same time.

ONCE THE PORT IS IN PLACE

You can feel port. It is usually not flush with the body and can stick out a bit. The nurse uses a needle to poke through the skin into the reservoir to access the port.

Before leaving the house on the day of chemotherapy, Michael would use Emla® cream, a numbing cream that he would place over the port site. We would then put plastic wrap over the area that had cream on it. The plastic wrap serves as a barrier so you don't stain your shirt; at the same time it aids in the cream's absorption. By the time Michael would get to his appointment for his chemotherapy, the port area would be numbed, so when they stuck him with the needle he didn't feel it. Also, if you have a port, you are going to want to wear either a shirt that buttons up the front or one that is lower cut. This way the nurse has easy access to the port, and you feel more comfortable.

When the nurse is accessing the port, he or she should be wearing gloves and a mask to prevent infection. After accessing the port with a needle and making sure it is working properly, the nurse will hook up the infusion line. Then he or she will put a large square piece of tape over the top of it to keep it in place. This way the needle won't just pop out of the reservoir inadvertently.

BENEFITS

One of the main benefits of a port is that you don't have to get your blood drawn from a peripheral vein using an IV needle type device. Not only are you going to be getting chemotherapy, you have to have blood drawn for the lab results. So you're going to get poked multiple times on several occasions. If you have a port, it's easier and more comfortable.

It also makes it easier for the professional staff to draw blood. If they can't find your veins, it could cause a delay of therapy. You definitely do not want to have to delay therapy just because the staff cannot access your veins.

With a port, you also have a decreased risk of what we call "estravasation." Estravasation is when the IV medication is administered inadvertently into the tissue around the administration site. This can happen for a couple of reasons: it could be because the veins are brittle and the medication leaks out of the vein and into the surrounding area, or it could be because the needle is not quite positioned properly. Many chemotherapy drugs can be very caustic and cause pain, redness, and swelling if medication goes into the tissues inadvertently. However, chemotherapy medications that are classified as vesicants can do the most damage. Vesicants cause actual tissue necrosis (death) when administered outside of the vein. Depending on the type of chemotherapy medication you are going to be receiving, especially if it's very caustic or a vesicant, it might be advantageous to get a port.

RISKS

There are also risks involved in getting a port. Infection is the biggest risk from port placement and using a port. You will want to take all precautions to ensure that the area doesn't become infected, and to do this you will need to practice good port care. Keep the site clean. When the nurse accesses the port, he or she should be wearing gloves and a mask, and the port should be cleaned by the nurse prior to poking it with the needle. If it becomes red, swollen, or tender to the touch, you need to contact the physician. If the port becomes infected, they will give you antibiotics to treat it. In some cases, the port will need to be removed and replaced with another one. Infection prevention is the best practice; however, even with the best of care, they sometimes become infected.

Another problem that could occur is the formation of a clot around the tip of the port catheter. Often times the nurse can use medication to try to break up the small clot that is in there. This works quite often, but sometimes it doesn't. Sometimes a fibrin sheath forms in or around the port catheter area. A fibrin sheath is best thought of as a clump of cells that encase the catheter like a sock. This can allow blood to pool and then to clot. Furthermore, it can prevent medication from passing from the port catheter into the body. To ensure that the port is working, the nurse will check for a blood return by pulling a small amount of blood up with a syringe prior to using it to administer medication.

Additionally, there is a risk that the port catheter will come out of position. You may have to limit any activity that has anything to do with upper-body strengthening or with moving your arms above your head. This can cause the catheter to move back and forth and eventually out of place. So if you engage in lots of activity that requires the movement of your arms, you may have to limit it. Swimming is usually fine. Check with your doctor if you have questions about this.

Another downside, but not a risk, is that there is going to be a surgical scar. Physically, it will not cause any problems, so it can be overlooked as a drawback. However, psychologically, some people have difficulty being constantly reminded of all the things they went through during cancer treatment. Having a scar is a continual reminder of being or having been sick.

The port is removed the same way that it was placed inside the body; it's going to require a simple surgical procedure.

MICHAEL'S EXPERIENCE

Michael had a port placed and it worked really well for his chemotherapy. However, we did run into a couple of the problems related to the risk factors.

We were unaware of the risk that the port catheter could shift out of place with the movement of the arms over the head. Michael can be restless when sleeping. He sleeps with his arms over his head, cradling the pillow.

A couple of days before Thanksgiving, Michael called to tell me he had a kink in his neck. He figured that he had slept wrong and that there was nothing to worry about. Having separate houses, I didn't go to check on him until Thanksgiving. We were supposed to spend a quiet Thanksgiving together, just the two of us. When I got there, I saw that his neck was swollen. I tried to touch his neck, but he wouldn't let me. It was extremely sore. I told him that we needed to go to the hospital since he probably had a clot in his neck. Michael was refusing, so I called Dr. Kafri to inform him of the situation. He instructed us to go to the hospital. After much fussing by Michael, we finally went.

A resident took down Michael's history; however, he didn't do anything about the neck pain. When the ER physician overseeing the resident came in, he said he was going to discharge Michael. So I asked about what was going to be done about the swollen neck and neck pain. I told him that Michael had a port, and that we were instructed by his oncologist to come in to see if it was a clot.

I'm not sure what was communicated by the resident to the ER physician because he seemed surprised by this. The physician tried to examine Michael's neck, but Michael was in so much pain that he wouldn't allow the physician to touch it. The doctor then decided to do a CT scan of his neck and chest, which would allow them to see the port and catheter placement. They found that the catheter had actually looped up in into his jugular, so they admitted him to the hospital. Dr. Kafri wanted the surgeon to save the port if possible. Michael had already received his scheduled six cycles of chemotherapy, but he still needed to receive his trial medication, Zevlin®.

At first, we were told that Michael's catheter had come out of place. Instead of the catheter following a straight line to the heart, it formed a loop in his jugular. This was what the doctors thought was causing the neck pain and phlebitis. The next day when Dr. Kafri came to check on Michael, he showed us the CT scan results of the looped catheter. When going through the CT images, Dr. Kafri noticed that it looked like a clot had formed in the looped area of the catheter. A test called a "Doppler" was ordered. The Doppler showed that a clot had formed around the catheter and loop, which meant that the port catheter could not be repositioned back into place and was going to have to be removed. The blood thinners Heparin® and Coumadin® were then given to allow the body to work on breaking up the clot. Michael was on the Coumadin® for six weeks afterward, but the clot never did quite dissolve. His body ended up dissolving the area around the clot and redirecting blood flow to other veins in the neck. Even though Michael had complications, getting a port placed for his chemotherapy was still the right decision.

PICC LINE

Another option for medication delivery is a PICC line. PICC stands for peripherally inserted central catheter. It is like a central line catheter, like a port, in the sense that the catheter tip is near your heart and can remain in place for a month or longer. With the help of ultrasound, the line is threaded into a large vein of your upper arm until the tip is positioned close to the heart. Verification that the catheter tip is in the right place is done by a chest x-ray. The PICC line is usually inserted by a PICC nurse specialist, radiologist, or nurse practitioner. PICC lines can have single, double, or multiple lumens, which look like tubes that stick out of your arm.

Different medications can be inserted into the body through them. If you have a multiple-lumen PICC, more than one medication can be run at a time through the separate lumens, as long as the medications are compatible.

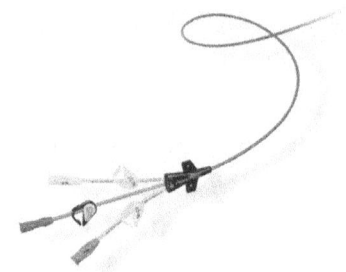

MULTIPLE-LUMEN PICC LINE[3]

ADVANTAGES OF PICC LINES

There are a couple of advantages to having a PICC line placed. The first advantage is that the nurse won't have to try to search for IV access. The other advantage is, just like a port, the medication will stay in the PICC until it reaches the catheter tip near the heart where it mixes with a large volume of blood. This ensures less risk of phlebitis or irritation of the vein with caustic drugs like chemotherapy.

POTENTIAL PROBLEMS WITH PICC LINES

As with ports, there are some risk factors associated with PICC lines, including infection at the site where the catheter enters the vein. You need to contact the physician if you see any redness or swelling around the PICC line. The line can cause phlebitis, which is an inflammation of the vein. PICC lines also have the risk of thrombus, which is a clot. This can either occur in the vein itself or in the catheter.

All in all, though, port placements and PICC lines are great ways to get chemotherapy infused.

"The courage of life is often a less dramatic spectacle than the courage of the final moment; but it is no less a mixture of triumph and tragedy."
John F. Kennedy

CHAPTER 6

PHYSICAL EFFECTS OF CANCER, CHEMOTHERAPY, AND TREATMENT

There is a wide range of physical effects resulting from cancer, chemotherapy, and support treatment. While not an exhaustive list, this chapter includes the most common side effects of chemotherapy. You may not experience all of the listed physical effects, but these are the most prevalent.

NAUSEA AND VOMITING

The one of the side effects that concerns most people is nausea and vomiting. When I first started working in oncology, the antiemetic medications that targeted chemotherapy-induced nausea were new on the scene. Prior to that time, no medications were available to combat it. As a result, people often became very sick from their treatment. There is still the fear of nausea and vomiting today, but now we have several medications in our arsenal to alleviate this problem.

It is important to try to prevent the nausea and vomiting. First of all, the nausea is a very uncomfortable feeling, and the vomiting can lead to dehydration. Dehydration can lead to hospitalization to replenish IV fluids and electrolytes that are lost from vomiting.

When it comes to nausea, one of the most appropriate metaphors is a freight train. Just as a freight train is easier to stop before, or right as, it is leaving the station, so is nausea. If you address the nausea when it first begins, it will be easier to stop and control it. If you let it go on, it becomes more difficult to control, and this can then lead to vomiting. Your freight train is now barreling along a mile down the track and more difficult to stop. So you will want to stop it in the beginning.

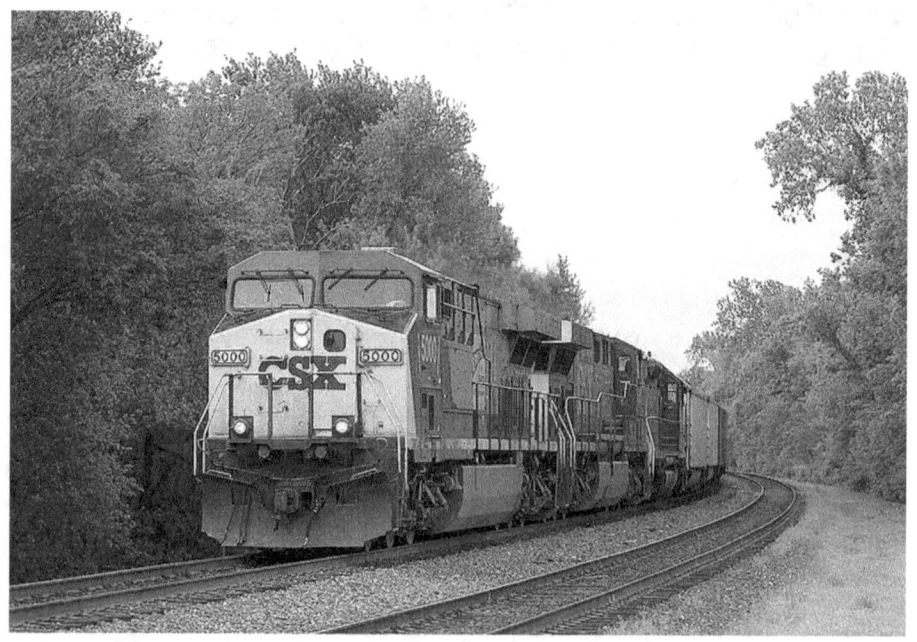

FREIGHT TRAIN[4]

When Michael had his first chemotherapy, he was given an anti-nausea medication, Aloxi®, in the IV line. He was also given another anti-nausea medication to take orally on the days following chemotherapy. The day after chemotherapy the nausea was really bad. He had taken one medication, Compazine®, and it wasn't helping him. So he wanted to just go lie down. I told him that he couldn't and that we had to call the doctor right away because the anti-nausea medication they were giving him was not working. We needed to use something else.

There are many medications for nausea. If the one that you're using is not working, there are others available. Call your doctor if the medication or medications that you've been given are not effective.

We called the oncologist, and he called in a prescription for another medication, Zofran®. It was helpful in stopping the nausea for Michael, which was good because his nausea was pretty bad. He had to take it after every chemo session twice a day for a week. There was no getting around the taking of Zofran®, as we did not want the nausea to become uncontrollable, which could have led to vomiting.

Because Michael was still having some problems with nausea, we also tried another anti-nausea medication, Emend® in the IV formulation. I wanted it to be given intravenously because then it would be completely covered by the insurance. Emend® also comes in an oral form, but Michael would have had to pay the co-pay for it. This shows that knowing your insurance coverage may save you additional money. In the end, though, the medication did not seem to provide greater nausea control and actually caused increased constipation. So we did not use it again.

CHANGES IN TASTE AND SMELL

Tied in with the nausea is the lack of desire to eat. Besides simply not feeling well, you will experience a lot of taste changes, which happen as a result of the taste buds being affected by the chemotherapy. Some smells become intolerable and may even cause you to become nauseous. To combat this, eat food that is mostly bland. Avoid spicy foods; you will probably be unable to tolerate them anyway.

With regard to smells, use unscented soaps and ask others to refrain from wearing perfume or cologne. Additionally, some foods will also smell terrible.

CONSTIPATION

Another common side effect of receiving chemotherapy is constipation, which can be caused by a couple of things. A major source of constipation can be the anti-nausea medications; that's unfortunately one of their side effects. Anti-nausea medications stop the peristaltic wave, which goes up from the stomach and into the esophagus to prevent nausea. But they also prevent peristalsis of things coming out on the other end. This leads to constipation. Additionally, some chemotherapy medications themselves can be constipating, so you might get a double whammy when it comes to this kind of discomfort.

The recommendation that the physician will usually give is to increase your fiber intake; however, that recommendation might be slightly difficult to follow. Sometimes just eating can be a challenge. Most of the time, though, you will be put on medication for the constipation. There several over-the-counter medications on the market you can use. Miralax® is a popular choice, and Senna-S® also works well. *The constipation can become severe*, so make sure you are taking this medication!

DIARRHEA

On the flip side, you could also experience diarrhea. Some chemotherapy can cause diarrhea as a side effect. Antidiarrheal medicine is used for this problem and to prevent dehydration. As I said earlier, dehydration can lead to hospitalization, so it is very important to prevent the loss of fluids and electrolytes. You really need to keep this under control. If the antidiarrheal medication is not working, you need to call your physician.

If you have any history of Crohn's disease, ulcerative colitis, or irritable bowl, the oncologist will probably opt to use other chemotherapy agents. This is why it is always important to give a medical history that is as full and accurate as possible.

FATIGUE

Fatigue is a very common side effect of chemotherapy. However, it is not only a result of chemotherapy, but also of the disease in and of itself. Growing tumors consume a lot of energy to keep up their pace of expansion. Prior to diagnosis, Michael was extremely fatigued and even had bouts of exhaustion.

When the fatigue is caused by the chemotherapy, it can be because of low blood counts. Specifically, exhaustion can be the result of low hemoglobin. Hemoglobin is the component of the red blood cell that contains iron and transports oxygen throughout the body.

When hemoglobin is low, the physician may opt to give you a blood transfusion in order to raise its level. Additionally, there is medication that can be used to raise the blood counts if they are too low.

Also be aware that if you take iron tablets or multi-vitamins that contain iron, they can cause constipation.

Because fatigue can be due to the chemotherapy, the cancer, and the low blood counts, it is *not* relieved by rest or sleep. Even so, you will be doing just that—sleeping. After the second or third cycle of chemotherapy, you could feel even more fatigued or completely exhausted.

Fatigue is one of the main reasons why you assembled your personal team in the first place. Call them into action for the tasks you agreed upon in the initial meeting. Whatever the task is that the person agreed to do, whether it was housework, yard work, cooking, running errands, paying bills, and so on, it is at this point that you're going to need him or her to help you take care of work you're unable to do. If you don't have a personal team assembled, check with the cancer resource center for free or low-cost help that may be available.

INFECTION

You want to minimize your risk of infection. In order to do this, you are going to want to limit your exposure to things or people that could make you sick. If your family or friends are sick, tell them that they can't come over to visit.

In order to minimize the risk of becoming infected, you are going to want to know when your nadir from chemotherapy is going to occur. Your nadir is when the blood levels (white blood cells, red blood cells, and platelets) drop to their lowest point. Generally, most nadirs occur within seven to ten days, and it is at this time you are most susceptible to infection. The white blood cells are divided into several types of cells, and specifically, neutrophils are the ones that help you to fight off infection. You may be instructed to take a medication that is designed to increase your white count when it is low, which may coincide with the time of your nadir. Sometimes, medication is given prophylactically (for prevention) if your chemotherapy regimen is known to dramatically drop the white blood count.

You *must* have a thermometer. Purchase one if you don't have one, because if you develop a fever, you *have* to call the oncologist with your temperature. If you have a Health Care Reimbursement or Health Care Savings account, thermometers are covered under these plans.

At your first oncologist visit, he or she should have told you at what temperature you should call. Make sure to write this down and have it for reference.

At any point in your cycle of treatment, and especially at the nadir time, you run the risk of having a low white blood cell count. If your white blood count is low, you won't have a normal immune system to fight infection. Therefore, if you have a temperature and a low white count, you're going to be hospitalized so you can receive the required antibiotics.

LOW PLATELETS

Platelets are cells in the blood that are responsible for hemostasis. Hemostasis is the process which causes bleeding to stop in a damaged vein and the process of clot formation.

Chemotherapy can lower the platelet count, which can affect the amount of time it takes your blood to clot. This could potentially lead to increased bleeding. Because of this, your physician may instruct you to avoid taking aspirin or NSAIDS (non-steroidal anti-inflammatory drugs such as Ibuprofen), as these products can also increase the time it takes your blood to clot. Be sure to ask the physician if you should avoid these while you are on a chemotherapy regimen.

Because of increased bleeding potential, you should use a soft bristle toothbrush and an electric razor.

Contact your physician immediately if you have any excessive bruising or bleeding.

MOUTH SORES

You may experience mouth sores because chemotherapy affects rapidly dividing cells, and the mouth is full of them, making it particularly vulnerable. Because mouth sores can occur at any time without warning, make sure to use a mouthwash without alcohol. Alcohol will burn and make the mouth sores even more painful. Michael used Biotène® oral rinse. If you do end up developing mouth sores, there are some liquid swish-and-spit medications available to help soothe and heal the sores.

As part of his chemotherapy treatment, Michael had a medication called doxorubicin, which makes you more susceptible to developing mouth sores. There has been some literature stating that using ice chips and cold water while the doxorubicin is being administered may help decrease or prevent mouth sores. This is because the blood is shunted away from the mouth area while the medication is being given. As a result, the medication may be prevented from going into the cells and therefore not affect them as much. It may or may not work for you, but it seemed to work for Michael because when he used the ice chips, he didn't get mouth sores. However, the one time that he did not use ice chips and cold water while getting the doxorubicin, he did develop them.

THRUSH

Thrush is a fungus that grows in the mouth and throat. It appears as a white coating on your tongue, mouth, and/or throat. The fungus appears because your immune system isn't strong enough to prevent it from growing inside you.

If you see thrush, you will want to call the physician immediately and get it treated. There is IV and oral medication available to combat it. The oral medication is in a swish-and-swallow liquid to coat the affected area and kill the fungus.

COGNITIVE CHANGES

There will most likely be some cognitive changes in the person getting chemotherapy. Cognitive changes affect such things as memory, understanding, and reasoning, and they can happen before, during, and possibly continue for years after receiving the chemotherapy. These mental changes are sometimes referred to as "chemo brain." Because these changes can actually occur before chemo even begins, "chemo brain" may not be the most accurate term. However, it is still commonly used to refer to these changes.

With these changes, you can experience forgetfulness, and sometimes you will feel like you're in a fog. When in this state of fogginess, you will be unable to concentrate and recall things easily. Because of this, you need to write things down and receive support in the areas that need detailed attention. For example, with Michael, his bills were on automatic bill pay. However, there was an "extra" charge he forgot about, which was his yearly renewal fee. Because things were on automatic pilot, it took several months before we discovered that the renewal charge put him over his account limit that month. In addition to this, the balance was not being completely paid each month, which meant that he ended up incurring additional interest and overage charges.

You may also experience forgetfulness with regard to simple tasks such as taking your medication. Did you take it? Did you not take it? Recording things at the time you are actually doing them is helpful. It is best to have a calendar of when and which medications to take. In the office at St. Joseph, the nurses make up a calendar with all the anti-nausea medications, steroids, and other medications the person may be on after chemotherapy and before the next appointment. Your calendar should include office visits, lab visits, and any other follow-up testing that is needed.

You may experience trouble remembering common words. Michael would be talking and forget simple, everyday words. He would end up pointing to an object, such as a chair, because he could not remember its name. It was as if the word was on the tip of his tongue, but he couldn't recall it. I would say the word once I realized what he was trying to articulate. He would then thank me and say the word himself before we would continue with the conversation. He would feel less frustrated if I first said the word; then he could say it back to me. Once the chemotherapy was completed, the verbal memory problem decreased significantly.

Michael also felt like he was losing his mental faculties at times. This can be very frightening and evoke many emotions, including frustration, anger, depression, and so forth. Being not only physically sick, but additionally experiencing these mental changes can be overwhelming. However, it is not uncommon to experience these side effects. Considering that other people might notice this change in you, it may be less stressful if you let others know that it is a common side effect of the disease and/or treatment.

If you try to multitask, it could be very difficult; therefore, it is best to do one thing at a time. As a result, you will be more successful in accomplishing the task.

PERIPHERAL NEUROPATHY

Peripheral neuropathy is numbness of the extremities such as the feet and fingers and can be caused by some chemo medications. Peripheral neuropathy can be either permanent or transient. There are medications available to reduce the severity of the peripheral neuropathy if you do experience it.

Michael's was transient. After the first cycle of R-CHOP, which has vincristine as part of the regimen, Michael experienced numbness of the ring and pinky fingers on his left hand that radiated up about an inch or two above his wrist. In his follow-up visit, we told his oncologist about it. Dr. Kafri decided to continue the medication as prescribed since the peripheral neuropathy was not severe. By the end of the second cycle, Michael no longer experienced any peripheral neuropathy.

If you're diabetic, you will want to talk with your oncologist about receiving medications that can possibly cause peripheral neuropathy. The oncologist may change the kind of medication he or she prescribes or may reduce the dose to try to prevent peripheral neuropathy from occurring. If you already have peripheral neuropathy due to diabetes, you should have an in-depth discussion with your doctor about whether or not you should be put on such medication.

INTOLERANCE TO HEAT AND COLD

It is not uncommon to develop intolerance to heat or cold. Before Michael's diagnosis, he loved to be in cooler temperatures. There was always a fan going in our bedroom! After chemotherapy, we sometimes had to set the thermostat at eighty-five degrees Fahrenheit for him to stop shivering.

Hormone therapies can often cause hot flashes. In general, people receiving hormone medication can feel very hot and flushed. Also, after treatment is completed, heat or cold intolerance can remain.

HAIR LOSS

Not all kinds of chemotherapy cause hair loss, but a large percentage of them do. If you want to wear a wig, consult your chemo resource center for recommended places to buy them. Some hospitals even provide haircutting and wig-fitting consultations on the premises. Some people prefer to just wear caps or do-rags instead. When Michael lost his hair during chemo, he wore a cap. After his chemotherapy cycles were complete, his hair grew back thicker and darker. When hair grows back after chemotherapy is finished, it can often be thicker, darker, and curlier.

If you would like to try to prevent your hair from falling out, there is a company (www.PenguinColdCaps.com) that has invented "cold cap" therapy. Cold cap therapy uses a cap that cools the hair follicles during chemotherapy infusion. This may prevent the hair follicles from becoming damaged and thus minimizing hair loss.

PAIN

There can be pain associated with cancer, and this is usually due to tumor pain. Whether the cancer is local or has spread to other parts of the body, the pain can become severe. Do not suffer through it. Some patients try to be brave and soldier through it. Others are concerned about becoming addicted to the pain medication. I repeat: *do not* suffer through the pain. Always tell your oncologist about the location of your pain and its severity.

Many pain medications also can cause constipation, so make sure you are taking medication for constipation if you experience any symptoms.

STEROIDS

Steroids can be used as part of your regimen. They are usually used to prevent nausea, and sometimes high- dose steroids are used to help the chemotherapy work. They are going to make you hungry, and this, in turn, can lead to weight gain. They also will make you crave sugar and retain water. Therefore, you will want to eat natural sugars such as fruit and avoid refined sugars. Additionally, you will want to avoid salt.

In our situation, I tried to get all the sugar out of the house because I knew Michael would always crave it. However, his family would sneak him cookies and brownies. This really upset me, but at some point I had to give in. There was just so much going on. Considering everything else that was happening, I ended up giving in a little bit on this. But I would still tell him that he really should not be eating the sweets. Overall, Michael did gain weight during the course of his chemotherapy. In the beginning, he actually lost weight because he was unable to eat, but as time went on, he ended up gaining weight.

CHEMO ELIMINATION

Most chemotherapy medications are largely eliminated through the urine. You are going to need to drink *a lot* of water to flush out the chemotherapy medication. Otherwise, it may cause more undesirable side effects and adversely affect the healthy cells in your body.

As part of his regimen, Michael received doxorubicin, which is red in color. For two days after the chemotherapy, his urine was red. If you receive doxorubicin, be aware that your urine could be reddish or orangey in color.

Because you're going to be eliminating the chemotherapy compound through your urine and bodily fluids, you will want to keep your pets and small children away from the toilet and especially from playing in it or drinking its water. Otherwise, they may become exposed to the chemotherapy medication that you are eliminating. For safety, flush twice after using the toilet. Also, during this time, men should sit on the toilet when urinating instead of standing.

In regard to sexual intimacy with your partner, use the information you got from the oncologist. If your oncologist recommended condom use, remember to purchase them. Otherwise, abstain from sex for the recommended time frame.

FLUID RETENTION

Even though you need to drink a lot of water to eliminate the chemotherapy, you could end up retaining fluid. You could also experience pitting edema in your extremities, which is when you push down with your thumb on the area that has the fluid, and the indentation from where the thumb pushed down remains.

Additionally, fluid retention could develop in the abdomen or chest area of your body. To eliminate the fluid retention, the oncologist may put you on medication, and if there is a lot of fluid, he or she may have to physically drain it. With fluid retention in general, but especially when edema is present in the abdomen or chest area, you may experience shortness of breath and/or difficulty breathing. If this happens, contact your oncologist immediately.

Because Michael's edema was in his legs, we first tried compression stockings. However, they never fit well and would roll down frequently. They also caused his toes to become purple when he wore them. So Dr. Kafri put him on the medication Lasix® to help him get rid of the excess water.

KEEPING TRACK

To make the process of keeping track easier, additional aids are listed below. Start by writing in your chemotherapy regimen. Then, investigate! Get all the information you can about the chemotherapy and support medications prescribed, including their side effects and any recommended support care. To find out the specific side effects you may experience from your chemotherapy regimen, go to www.chemocare.com and click on "drug information." Support care information is also available on the website.

Your Chemotherapy Regimen:
Your specific chemo regimen is _____
Frequency: _____
This regimen has the following medications:
    1. _____
    2. _____
    3. _____
    4. _____
    5. _____
    6. _____

Your anti-nausea medications are:

1. _____
2. _____
3. _____

Your support medications are:

1. _____
2. _____
3. _____

For example:

Michael's regimen: R-CHOP

Frequency: Every twenty-one days

His regimen had the following medications:

1. Rituximab
2. Doxorubicin
3. Cyclophosphamide
4. Vincristine
5. Prednisone

Michael's anti-nausea medications were:

1. Aloxi®—given on the day of chemotherapy
2. Zofran®—oral medication taken twice a day for one week after chemotherapy

Michael's support medications were:

1. Senna-S® – oral medication taken for constipation
2. Ativan® –oral medication taken for anxiety or sleep as needed

After receiving chemotherapy:

- Write down your side effects.
- Call the oncologist if the side effects are intolerable.
- Take the list of the side effects that you experienced to your next doctor's appointment.

Remember to get a journal in which to write down all of your physical changes, and take it to your next appointment. Copy the chemotherapy regimen template and note additional questions in your journal to discuss with your oncologist.

"The beginning of knowledge is the discovery of something we do not understand."
Frank Herbert

CHAPTER 7

MALNUTRITION KILLS

According to the National Cancer Institute's website, anorexia, defined as the loss of appetite or desire to eat, is typically present in 15 to 25 percent of all cancer patients at the stage of diagnosis.[5] In addition to this, it can occur as a side effect of chemotherapy treatments. Anorexia can also speed up the process of cachexia.

Cachexia is a progressive wasting syndrome that manifests as the loss of body weight, fat, and muscle, as well as in the form of generalized weakness. Cachexia is estimated to be the immediate cause of death in 20 to 40 percent of cancer patients, and it can develop in individuals who appear to be eating adequate amounts of calories and protein.[6] However, cachexia often will occur in people who have tumor-related issues that prevent the maintenance of fat and muscle. Those who have the greatest risk of developing cachexia are people diagnosed with gastrointestinal-tract cancers.

The process of developing cachexia is explained further by Keith I. Block, MD, medical/scientific director of the Block Center for Integrative Cancer Treatment in Skokie, Illinois: "The current scientific consensus is that cancer cachexia results primarily from an underlying metabolic imbalance induced by the cancer, causing the body's metabolism to speed up. The malignancy generates the production of low-grade inflammatory molecules that break down lean muscle and can disrupt immune functioning. The heavy consumption of fats, refined flours, and sugars found in the traditional American diet can increase this inflammation, contributing to a lack of appetite, a more debilitating weight loss, and actually promote the very disease the patient is trying to fight."

WHAT TO EAT

In order to get a better handle on your nutrition, you should shop in the outside aisles of the grocery store, not the inside ones. In the outside aisles, you're going to find fresh fruits and vegetables, lean meats, and dairy products. Because of the risk of cachexia, many oncologists recommend increasing the consumption of lean protein. Check with the oncologist and/or nutritionist about the specific recommendations.

The inside aisles of the grocery store are where you will mostly find processed foods. These are the items to stay away from. For example, try replacing traditional desserts that are heavy in flour, fats, and sugars with fresh fruit.

However, there is a slight modification in your thinking that you will need to make. In the past, it was often recommended that you avoid raw fruits and vegetables because of the bacteria on the produce that could make you very susceptible to infection. Now it is advised to thoroughly wash the fruits and vegetables if you want to eat them. If your family or friends are providing meals for you, let them know this information. Still, you should avoid ordering raw produce when eating out. Of course, cooking fruits and vegetables will kill the bacteria on their exterior.

Michael would experience anorexia after his chemotherapy. The only foods he could tolerate eating were those that were not spicy whatsoever. They had to be very bland. For about five days after chemotherapy, he would eat ground turkey and small yellow baked potatoes, and that's about it.

The way to combat the anorexia is to eat small, frequent meals. This will also help with any nausea you might be experiencing.

Having a little bit of something in your stomach will keep it settled, and you'll be less likely to be nauseous while you continue to get your calories. And most likely, you're not going to want to eat a large meal. It is just not going to be appealing.

On many occasions, Michael would not want to eat, so I had to bargain with him. I would say to Michael, "Just eat *half* of this quarter of the potato." Out of a small yellow potato that was about two inches in diameter, he would eat a quarter of it. From a half-pound of ground turkey, he would eat one-tenth of it. I would always try to get a bit of something into him, and then, a few hours later, I would try to get him to eat a little bit more of it. If he wasn't up to it, I would try something else that was more appealing to him at the time. The food had to have very little fat and no spice; otherwise he would find it very nauseating.

Another way to get calories and protein is to use supplements. Both Boost® and Ensure® make liquid and bar supplements. You can use a blender to mix the liquid product with fruit or yogurt to add extra nutrients.

After a couple rounds of chemotherapy, Michael started to regain his appetite. When he was on steroids, he would crave cookies, cakes, and brownies. His family would sneak in desserts because they knew that I didn't want him to have them. But the reason I forbade these foods wasn't solely because of the weight gain from empty calories; it was also because these foods could be detrimental to his recovery. This often led to fights, but at some point I had to let it go. The family would occasionally bring him dessert, and I just expressed that I didn't think that it was a good idea for him to eat those things.

Having been on steroids myself, I can understand how they can be a very powerful factor in the craving of food in general. My advice would be to try to satisfy the craving by eating something healthy like fruit instead of processed desserts.

If you have loved ones who are going to be cooking for you, let them know that you prefer not to have processed foods. Ask them also to cook foods that would be appealing to the person getting chemotherapy, and keep a journal of what is appealing what is not appealing or tolerable. This way, the people cooking for you will get an idea of what they might prepare.

ANTIOXIDANTS

Within this discussion of nutrition, there is a gray, almost paradoxical, area when it comes to the consumption of antioxidants. Cancer can arise from oxidative stress cause by free radicals, and antioxidants can help prevent cancer by neutralizing free radicals. However, your oncologist may advise you to limit or eliminate foods and supplements that contain antioxidants from your diet. It is thought that antioxidants can interfere with the chemotherapy by reducing its efficiency in killing the cancer. This is because chemotherapy kills cancer by producing free radicals that damage the DNA of the cancer cells. When the DNA becomes damaged, the cell has a difficult time repairing itself. If it cannot repair itself, the cell dies.

Concerning antioxidant use, more information is needed about the consumption of high-dose IV ascorbic acid (vitamin C). There is some evidence that high doses of intravenous vitamin C may eradicate cancer. This leads to many other questions about the use of antioxidants in cancer patients that, at present, do not have clear answers.

With Michael, I would eliminate the foods that contained antioxidants for about one week after he received chemotherapy. His chemotherapy agents were eliminated within a couple days, and the nadir time was about ten days. When I knew that the chemotherapy was out of his system and had done its job, I added antioxidants, such as oranges and blueberries, back into his diet.

It is important to find out what the elimination time is for your chemotherapy because your oncologist will most likely want you to remove antioxidant foods and supplements at least for that period of time. He or she may want to eliminate the antioxidants even up to the nadir time. Check with your oncologist to see what he or she recommends.

"Life is like a roller coaster. There are many ups and downs with very few flat spots."
Stephanie Carrothers

CHAPTER 8

EMOTIONAL EFFECTS

This journey through cancer treatment can have a lot of emotional effects, and they can take a toll everyone going through this experience. You will most likely experience a "roller coaster" of emotions. Typically, anxiety and depression will be associated with receiving the diagnosis, along with a lot of anger and disbelief that this is happening. Remember to seek professional help if necessary.

ANXIETY

Sometimes anxiety can creep up on you, and you might not recognize it at first. This happened to Michael on his way to one of his chemotherapy appointments. When I came to pick up Michael for his chemotherapy, I didn't recognize that he was anxious; he didn't seem any different than the other times I had picked him up. However, as we were driving, he started yelling at me to slow down. We were still in the residential zone by the house, so I was only going twenty-five miles per hour. When I told him how fast I was going, he looked at the speedometer and settled down a bit. However, when we got on the freeway, he again started yelling at me not to drive so fast. I was in the right lane and doing fifty-five. When I explained this to him, he looked again at the speedometer while I pointed out that people were passing me on the left side. Michael said that it felt like we were doing ninety.

When we got to the cancer center, the typical routine was to first go to the lab and get blood drawn, and then go see the physician. At that point, I didn't think much about Michael's state, but as the day continued, he became more and more agitated. After seeing the physician, we went to the infusion room. By this time, he had become extremely agitated. I asked the nurse if she could call the physician for an order for some Ativan®, an anti-anxiety medication. Michael normally took it at home in tablet form. However, we had left it at home. The nurse was able to get an order from the oncologist for the IV form of the medication. I advise carrying anti-anxiety medication with you at all times if you have it prescribed because the anxiety can come out of nowhere, and it's best to always have something on hand.

Anxiety can be a normal response to receiving treatment, and it is very common in people coming in for the first chemotherapy treatment. The fear of the unknown coupled with the diagnosis can be overwhelming. If you experience these emotions, tell your oncologist.

DEPRESSION

Typically, anxiety and depression are connected. Mild antidepressants may be prescribed if you are experiencing depression, so talk openly with your oncologist about your feelings.

ANGER AND DEFIANCE

There can be a lot of anger regarding the diagnosis and cancer symptoms. I have seen patients become extremely angry, especially those who believed they did everything right when it came to diet and exercise, yet they still developed cancer.

Additionally, people can become angry about losing their health, both physically and cognitively. As a caregiver, you cannot take your loved one's anger personally. You need to realize that it is coming from a fear of total loss.

Michael wasn't angry as much as he was defiant. I like to refer to this as the "I don't want to do this and you can't make me" behavior.

Many times Michael didn't want to go to his chemo appointments. Who could blame him? I sure didn't. He was going to get treatment that was going to make him feel like hell for three weeks, and just when he was beginning to feel better, he would have to go back in for the next round. I can understand him not wanting to go. On one occasion, though, he was really refusing to go, and he stomped around the house like a three-year-old, declaring that he was not going and that I couldn't make him. I told him that he was going to go, and I pulled out all the logical reasons for him to do so. He just looked at me and stomped some more. Then he sat on the sofa with a look that said, "I dare you to make me." I told him we could do this the easy way or we could do it the hard way, and that he better not make me break out my martial arts. At this, we both laughed, and he joked about me beating up a poor cancer patient. Once we started laughing, it broke the tension, and we could be on our way. We were a bit late for his appointment, but we still made it in time for him to be treated.

When difficult situations arise, try to lighten the mood with laughter. It breaks the tension. Laughter truly is the best medicine.

WITHDRAWAL

Cancer patients also frequently experience emotional withdrawal and the desire to become reclusive. The patient can start to feel like staying inside and withdrawing from society, family, and friends. The feeling of not wanting to go out and do things can begin to take over. Becoming a hermit can be appealing, because the person doesn't feel good, doesn't want to deal with questions or looks from other people, is fatigued, and/or is tired of putting up a brave front.

If you are the loved one seeing this happen, it is best to help by encouraging the person to take small trips with you. Pick an activity that is not too long and has a flexible ending point. For example, choose a trip to the park instead of going to see a movie. When the person gets tired, you can always go back home at that moment. This way you have gotten the person out to get some fresh air and help change his or her mind-set.

EXERCISE

Exercise can help with some of these emotions. You don't have to have a full-on, intense workout. Just some moderate walking can help lift the mood.

"Sometimes we underestimate the influence of little things."
Charles W. Chesnutt

CHAPTER 9

CANCER PATIENT CAREGIVER

When your loved one receives the cancer diagnosis, it begins to sink in that you are going to be in this together for the long haul. This is going to be a marathon and not a sprint. A lot of questions begin to arise within you once you realize you will be dealing with a long-term diagnosis.

If your spouse or partner is the one who is diagnosed, what is your relationship like? This has the ability to bring you closer or tear you apart. If your relationship is already rocky, this period may prove to be very difficult. Having worked in oncology for quite some time, I have seen a multitude of reactions. Watching adversity bring people closer together, even when you couldn't believe that they could get any closer, is a beautiful thing to witness. For those who end up leaving their spouse or partner, there can be a tremendous amount of guilt surrounding that decision. Additionally, they may face the stigma of leaving someone in their time of need.

Regardless, even if your relationship is a good one, you're in for an emotional roller coaster. Your loved one could be angry, lost, depressed, anxious, or despondent in addition to being physically ill.

With Michael and I living apart, I would come help Michael out on the weekends and sometimes after work during the week. It was overwhelming. At times driving home, I would cry as different emotions welled up inside me. My feelings ranged from exhaustion to "This is hard," from "Why is this happening?" to "I hope that he gets better," and so forth. Different things and scenarios would run through my mind.

Because of this, you need to have a person you can talk to. If there is no one you know who you want to talk to about this, perhaps a professional would be the best bet. Sometimes we feel like we're burdening our friends with what we're going through. Maybe you think that they might not be able to understand. Perhaps you feel that they may be judgmental when you have seemingly selfish feelings such as wishing that the person would just be better so you didn't have to do everything, or being overwhelmed and feeling guilty that you can't do it all, or hoping that the person passes away, and everything in between.

An emotional support group with like-minded people who are experiencing the same thing can be very helpful. Check with your cancer resource center for support groups that are available.

A long-standing illness with your loved one can bring on depression and/or exhaustion. That's why it's so important to ask for help. As stated in the first chapter, you need to assemble a team to help you. These can be family members, friends, neighbors, or the community-service people, who are truly angels. They can help you with your needs. Allow others to help you. People do want to help; they feel that this allows them to contribute in some way to a situation in which they feel utterly helpless.

As for me, I am very proud person, and I like to do things myself. It was difficult to ask for help, but during that time, it was really necessary that I did ask. It can be humbling in its own right to realize that we can only do so much. It is through reaching out to others and allowing their help to be given and received that both the giver and receiver are strengthened.

Because I wanted to go to all of Michael's chemotherapy infusion and doctor's appointments, I was using up a lot of my PTO (paid time off) from work. As we were coming to the end of the chemotherapy cycles, I was running out of PTO, so I sent out an e-mail to my co-workers asking if any of them would give me eight to ten hours of their PTO so I could go to Michael's remaining appointments. I could have taken FLMA time, which is unpaid, and would have if I needed to go that route. However, thinking about the possibility of juggling finances was just another stress I didn't want to have to deal with. It was difficult to ask, but a person did donate PTO to my bank. I never knew who donated those hours to me. This is but one example of small ways that people can help you with what you need. If you need something, just ask.

If you are facing a long-standing illness and/or a long-standing treatment regimen, ask others to come to visit so you can take a break. You will need to have some personal time. Use this time to take a walk, or maybe go to church and pray, or perhaps see another friend for coffee or dinner. You need to have some time away from this diagnosis because it is going to be all-encompassing of your time. Therefore, you need to carve out a niche of time to recharge yourself. Take some time to do whatever rejuvenates you. Otherwise, you will become completely burned out. Burnout can be physical, emotional, spiritual, or any combination of the three.

When others come to visit, have a few guidelines set up for them to follow. Ask your family, friends, neighbors, and others who want to visit to have short, frequent visits instead of long, infrequent ones. Impress upon them that your loved one fatigues easily, if this is the case, necessitating shorter visits. Tell them to bring something else quiet to do if the person falls asleep such as crossword puzzles, knitting, a book, or their electronic device. Ask them the talk about what's happening out there in the world and to keep the conversation focused on positive things, avoiding a barrage of questions about how the individual is doing. If the person wants to share what is happening, he or she will. Catch the person up on what's going on with work or family. Bring pictures and notes for your loved one to look at after the visit so that they have something personal to remind them of the occasion. It can bring a smile when remembering what was talked about.

As a caregiver, be aware that people can feel uncomfortable visiting. When cancer is the diagnosis, and especially if your loved one has a lot of physical changes, it makes people uncomfortable because they are forced to face the person's mortality, as well as their own. Usually, we have our feelings about mortality neatly tucked away in the back of our mind. Bringing it to the forefront can make people uncomfortable and unsure of how to act. Just let them know that it's okay and that seeing your loved one can bring out different emotions in them. Sometimes you will end up being as much of a comforter to them as they are to you.

Be aware that people can say inappropriate things. One of the most common things is: "I know so-and-so who was diagnosed with (your type of cancer) and died." When Michael went into remission, guys he worked with started telling him he had the "fake" cancer. Sometimes people just do not know how to express their concern or feelings, while others feel like they need to say something profound. Unfortunately, some people will be so uncomfortable that they will no longer be present in your life.

"The months and years know what the days and weeks could never know."
Unknown

CHAPTER 10

OUTCOMES

A cancer diagnosis will eventually have an outcome. Because cancer is a serious, life-threatening disease, you should fill out an advance directive when you are diagnosed. This lets your family and medical staff know your wishes if you cannot speak for yourself. A fantastic, easy-to-understand document that is legal in forty-two states is the "Five Wishes®." Check your resource center for a copy of the document. If the center does not carry it, you can find it online at www.agingwithdignity.org.

REMISSION

The first outcome with your battle with cancer could be remission. Remission is when there's no evidence of cancer left in the body. At this point, there will be a follow-up schedule. You want to continue to follow up with your oncologist at the scheduled times, and if you were involved in a study, those appointments will probably be more often than if you were not. The more frequent appointment schedules are dictated by the guidelines of the study itself. If at any point you have symptoms between your follow-ups, you will want to call your oncologist right away so you can go in and get them checked out.

Be aware that some of the chemotherapy medications can leave lasting physical ailments. For example, Michael needs to lose some weight because of the doxorubicin that he received. Doxorubicin can weaken the heart muscle, and people who are overweight and have received doxorubicin are at greater risk of sudden cardiac death.

Other chemotherapies can cause peripheral neuropathy that sometimes cannot be reversed. Medications are available to make the neuropathy more tolerable. Other chemotherapies can cause a person to have sensitivity to cold. In the future, you could still have that sensitivity.

REMISSION FOLLOWED BY RECURRENCE

Remission followed by recurrence is the ultimate roller coaster of emotions. The initial cancer diagnosis brings out the fear of the unknown. Remission gives us the hope that we have beaten cancer. But for how long? When you go into remission, it is a state of cautious optimism. Recurrence could be just around the corner. When recurrence does occur, it brings more uncertainty. What is the next step? Will you have to have more chemotherapy? What side effects will that chemotherapy have? Will you go into remission again? These, along with other questions, will arise and have to be addressed. I highly recommend seeing a counselor at this point if you haven't previously. Recurrence can be a very low time both emotionally and spiritually.

STILL FIGHTING

Another outcome is that you will still be in the fight. Where I work, some cancer patients have been coming in for years. The treatment plan keeps the cancer at bay, but it doesn't put them into full remission. So they continue to come in according to their treatment plan.

Another outcome is that the person cannot overcome the cancer and dies while receiving hospice care or before going into hospice.

HOSPICE

Many family members feel that even talking about hospice is admitting defeat. There is a belief that hospice means losing hope when there still may be some type of cure. What needs to be realized is that the person did not give up; it is the body that has had enough. Even if the mind and spirit are willing, the body cannot be healed. Hope for a cure can be redefined as hope for the best quality of life for the time remaining.

To qualify for hospice, two conditions must be met. First, the physician has to state that the person is terminally ill and is not going to recover from his or her illness. Second, the person's life expectancy is less than six months. Hospice care is given wherever the person is residing, whether they're at home, in a nursing home, in the hospital, or, in some areas, in a hospice care center.

Hospice provides pain relief and management of symptoms. This is where treatment is not continued but comfort measures are maintained. Medication that would make the person more comfortable, such as pain medication, would be provided. Hospice care doesn't hasten death by withholding basic needs. Its purpose is to allow the person to be as comfortable as possible while providing the best quality of life.

"My mother is a big believer in being responsible for your own happiness. She always talked about finding joy in small moments and insisted that we stop and take in the beauty of an ordinary day. When I stop the car to make my kids really see a sunset, I hear my mother's voice and smile."
Jennifer Garner

CHAPTER 11

RIDING INTO THE SUNSET

It was January and the ground was covered in snow. As Michael and I were walking through the parking lot, Michael asked, "That's it? We're done?"

I shook my head yes.

"It's not going to come back?"

"That's what the doctor said. He thinks you will stay in remission." I smiled at him. Relief and exhaustion filled my body as I slid into the driver's seat.

"Yeah, but really? It's not coming back?" he asked again as he was climbing into the passenger side.

"You still have the follow-up appointments you have to go to." I said. But I knew what he was feeling. It was such an anticlimactic event. The struggles over the past months were so incredibly difficult, yet here we were walking out to the car as we had done so many other times before after appointments. After a pause I said with concern, "And if anything were to come up, we need to call him right away." My tone then became upbeat. "But, Dr. Kafri thinks you're in the clear!"

It was starting to sink in a bit more. We both smiled.

"Yay!" Michael exclaimed.

"Do you want to go out to dinner to celebrate?" I asked.

"No. I'm too tired. Maybe some other day." After a pause, he asked, "Is the tiredness ever going to go away?"

"It will probably be a few months before you feel like yourself again."

As we drove home, we talked about planning a trifecta party in the summer. We called it the *Michael's in Remission, We Got Married, Michael's Birthday* party. In June, family and friends came to honor the journey and celebrate life with us. The party was amazing. We laughed, conversed and were grateful. I even cried a bit.

What I learned most through all of this is to love and celebrate the life you have. Love is a verb and it expresses itself when it is shared. Remember that this is a marathon and not a sprint. So let people love you by helping you along the way. Whatever stage of your journey you find yourself in, whether you're in remission, still fighting, or entering hospice, my hope is that this information has equipped you for the best journey possible along the way.

With the support of others, you not only can survive but thrive through this process and make your own journey empowered and inspirational to those around you.

With much love-

Supplemental Information

Chapter 2
1 Oncotype DX testing for breast, prostate, and colon cancer. http://www.breastcancer.org/symptoms/testing/types/oncotype_dx

Chapter 4
Free download of Chapter 4 "Empowered Cancer Journey Journal" http://www.StephanieCarrothers.com

Chapter 6
Hair Loss Prevention: http://www.PenguinColdCaps.com
Side Effects & Support Care: http://www.chemocare.com

Chapter 10
Five Wishes: http://www.agingwithdignity.org.

REFERENCES

Chapter 5
2,3 Pictures © 2014 C.R. Bard, Inc. Used with permission. Bard, PowerPICC, and PowerPort are registered trademarks of C.R. Bard, Inc.

Chapter 6
4 Picture Used with permission by photographer Nate Beal http://www.flickr.com/photos/11370385@N03/2190453551

Chapter 7
5,6 "National Cancer Institute." *Nutrition in Cancer Care.* National Cancer Institute, 24 Oct. 2013.
http://www.cancer.gov/cancertopics/pdq/supportivecare/nutrition/healthprofessional

Additionally: Use of quoted material, permission granted by Keith I. Block, MD, medical/scientific director of the Block Center for Integrative Cancer Treatment in Skokie, Illinois

NOTES

NOTES

ABOUT THE AUTHOR

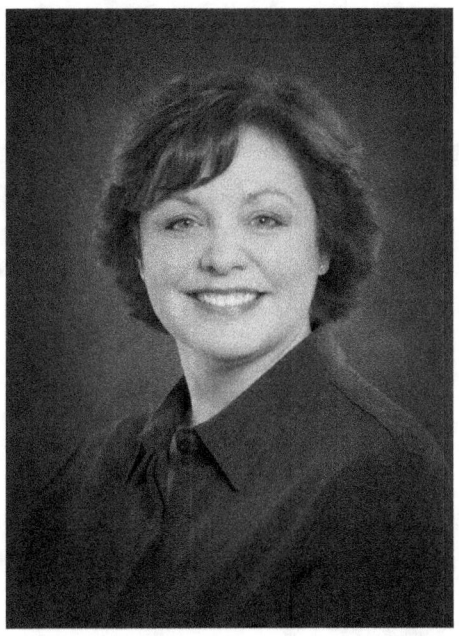

Stephanie Carrothers, RPh, graduated with a Bachelor of Science degree in Pharmacy from Wayne State University before dedicating the majority of her career to oncology. Her husband's diagnosis with lymphoma compelled her to write her first book, *Empowered Journey through Cancer.*

Stephanie Carrothers enjoys traveling with her husband, Michael, as well as hosting family game night and holiday meals at their home.